STAYING FIT
at work

The **Life Quality Management** series
for anyone balancing the needs of a
healthy lifestyle with the demands of
work. Each book can help you
improve the quality of your life, in
spite of work and its hazards.

Other titles include
Beating Stress at Work
Eating Well at Work
Surviving at Work

Penny Chorlton

Published in 1995

Health Education Authority
Hamilton House
Mabledon Place
London WC1H 9TX

ISBN 0 7521 0167 6

A CIP catalogue record for this book is available from the British Library.

The views expressed in this book are those of the author and not necessarily those of the Health
Education Authority.

The Publishers and Author have done their best to ensure the accuracy of all information in *Staying
Fit at Work*. However, they can accept no responsibility for any loss, illness, injury or inconvenience
sustained as a result of information or advice contained in the book.

Typesetting by Type Generation Ltd.

Printed in Great Britain by Biddles Ltd, Guildford, Surrey

Contents

Introduction

1	What is fitness?	1
2	How fit and active are you?	10
3	Why be fit?	20
4	Heart disease	27
5	Choosing the right exercise for you	37
6	Avoiding – and dealing with – injury	44
7	Excuses, excuses…	55
8	Problems and bad habits	62

Conclusions   74

Resources   77

Introduction

Given the choice, most people would rather be fit. The trouble is, though, that whatever job you do, and however much you earn, it's all too easy to put 'exercise' or 'physical activity' at the bottom of your list of priorities, either deliberately or unconsciously. The sad fact is that, for all but those in the most physically demanding types of occupations, most types of work are increasingly sedentary and, as we get older and more inactive, so we get inexorably fatter and more unfit.

This is a book for anyone who wants to put exercise and activity back into their lives, gradually and deliberately, so that they can enjoy life to the very fullest levels possible, whatever their age or present lifestyle.

However you decide to get moving, use the ideas in this book to have fun while you do it, and remember, the more you do, the more you'll want to do.

CHAPTER ONE

What is fitness?

The thought of getting fit can be all too daunting. Treadmills, cycling-machines, pulse monitoring, regular routines and so on ... they all give the general impression that the attempt to get fit is not going to be much fun.

True, some methods of getting fit can be tedious. But ask anyone who you know to be fit how they feel – and ask them to compare how they feel now compared to a time when they knew themselves *not* to be fit. It's virtually guaranteed that they will soon try and convert you to a fitter way of life.

Sadly, for most of the time, most of us are not fit. Although we may kid ourselves otherwise, secretly we know who we are! So be honest – are you fit?

How often does 'can't be bothered' cross your mind (and lips) when you know you have a strenuous task to do? It's not necessarily the task itself that is putting us off but the sheer effort required of us to sort out our desks, or take that outfit back to the shop, or spring-clean your bedroom. Even pleasant things like arranging to meet a friend for lunch may sometimes seem to be just too much effort.

Your lack of energy may be due to overwork. It is equally possible, though, that you are just feeling lethargic and inactive, and this is likely to permeate every aspect of your life, from work to play and all points in between.

The strange fact about fitness is that the more you do, the more you can do. People who are naturally active have a head start over those who are naturally more sluggish but everyone can speed up their own individual level of fitness simply by deciding that that is what they want to do.

THE THREE 'S'S

Fitness is made up of three components, known as the three 'S's. These are

- suppleness
- strength
- stamina.

Improving each aspect of fitness should be your overall goal, though you are probably already quite good in one or more aspect of fitness. Most of us fall down on the suppleness component which is unfortunate as this is the most important way in which we can avoid muscle strain or injury.

Suppleness

Suppleness or flexibility is crucial in our daily lives, whether we are at home or at work and whatever we do, at whatever age. We all need to be able to bend, stretch and balance, without risking serious injury and incapacity as a result.

As children, we are at our most flexible – just watch the way a toddler moves and bends, with a natural grace and automatically sensible posture. But as we get older, we tend to stiffen up, especially in the muscles that we don't use much. When we then try to use them in an unusual movement, such as reaching for something in a high cupboard or stretching out suddenly to catch a falling object, something can suddenly 'go' and we are in trouble...

Strength

Levels of strength are self-explanatory. We all have some degree of strength but there are tremendous variations from person to person.

Muscles need to be strong for us to be able to do things for ourselves. For example, we may need to be able to load and unload a trolleyful of shopping from the supermarket to the car and then into the house, or we may have to carry a tired child some distance, or we may have to move the furniture about.

Even if you are lucky enough to be able to employ others to do all your manual housework, you may want to be strong enough to have an ace serve in tennis or to spend a day on the golf course with the boss or colleagues – without risking a hernia.

Obviously we are all born with a pre-determined maximum level of strength – and most women will never achieve the level of strength of a six-foot man. All of us, however, can improve our capacity by exercising with weights. Muscular strength improves posture and support for your skeleton and healthy strong muscles also improve your body's shape and tone.

If your goal is primarily to improve your figure, reducing the flab alone won't be enough, you'll also need to do some abdominal exercises in order to tighten and strengthen the muscles in the tummy to hold it all in place!

Stamina

Stamina is required for rhythmic exercise such as walking, cycling and swimming. In addition to muscle strength, stamina requires a good capacity for oxygen delivery in the cardiovascular system and a strong capacity for work uptake in the muscles.

Stamina is important for those times when we have to summon up an extra physical effort. For example, you may have to visit an office which is situated on the fifth floor and the lift is out of order, or you may have to run to catch the train because you know that there won't be another one for at least two hours and your day will be ruined. While most of us can probably manage a quick sprint, many would have to sit down and recover for some time after such a strenuous exertion. Some of us would risk a heart attack, and a lot of us would take 15 minutes to reach that office and then need to recover for a similar length of time before being able to speak. Many of us would give up the attempt to catch that disappearing train!

MOST OF US ARE UNFIT

The most recent national survey of the state of fitness levels of the British population made startling reading. Although 80% of us declared that we felt we were fit, in fact two out of three men and half of all women were unable to perform a simple fitness test without getting out of breath or having to stop.

This involved over 1,500 adults who were asked to walk at a reasonable pace (about 3mph) both at ground level and then up a one in 20 slope. This was done for about 16 minutes or until each individual reached their personal target heart rate appropriate for their age. The results were noted (see below).

Researchers also found that only a tiny percentage – 14% of men and 4% of women, took part in regular weekly exercise, while less than a third engaged in any rigorous activity on a regular basis.

If you can't remember the last time you took any form of exercise, you are far from being alone. In fact, one in six people had not done anything vigorous enough to benefit their health in the week previous to being interviewed.

Among people over the age of 55, around a third never took part in any form of regular exercise .This is particularly worrying as middle-aged men are at the highest risk of coronary heart disease from other factors.

This study confirmed earlier findings in that there was a clear association between past participation in sport and the likelihood of developing heart disease, angina or breathlessness. Among the over 55s, 21% of men and 15% of women who had led inactive past lives suffered from one of these chronic conditions, compared with 14% and 3% respectively among men and women who had led active lives for most of the time, in the past.

The survey also found that those who had exercised regularly as children continued the practice into their adult years. Around 25% of those who said they were active teenagers were still leading relatively active lives compared with 2% who were currently active who admitted to being inactive when younger.

As far as people's working lives are concerned, routine physical activity plays a very minor role for most people. 90% of women and 80% of men said that their occupations did not involve them in any measurable degree of activity.

That's why you cannot assume that, just because you lead a busy life, you have a job and you are always tired and working against the clock, you are fit – far from it! It is precisely people like you who are most in need of doing something positive to get fitter.

Why are so many of us so unfit?

A lot of people are put off the whole idea of exercise because they just don't think of themselves as 'sporty'. But there's something much more fundamental to it than that – and that's summed up in just one word – SEDENTARY.

We have not always led such sedentary lives. Mass car-ownership, mass ownership of comprehensive home entertainment systems and a general shift away from manual labour to the push-button telecommunications era has meant that the vast majority of us can lead relatively inactive lives compared with even a generation ago.

And this change has affected our children too. Whereas in 1980 most children walked to and from school, now the vast majority go by bus or car, which means that neither they, nor the adults that might once have escorted them, take even a twice daily constitutional walk to and from the school gates.

Children are also less active when they get to school. Although physical education is now included in the national curriculum, the amount of time dedicated to PE and extra curricular activities varies greatly across the country. As a result, very early on in life before many of us even start work, regular sporting activity has ceased to play any part in our daily lives. The rot sets in very early.

Sir Roger Bannister, who ran the first four-minute mile, deplores the fact that so many schools have dropped sport. Exercise is a habit, like any other, and research shows that if you drop sport while you are young, you are less likely to incorporate it into your adult life. The reverse is also true, so you should aim to make sport and/or exercise just as much a part of your life as eating and sleeping.

Incredible as it may seem now, our grandfathers and great-grandfathers believed that we were all born with a set allotted lifespan and ration of energy. It was thought that the more vigorous a life you led, the more quickly you would burn up your allocated 'lot' and so people conserved their energy expenditure whenever they could.

Of course, for those generations, the sheer business of daily life was enormously physically taxing, with 'Shanks's pony' for transport, no cosy central heating, and vast amounts of manual labour expended by men and women alike going about their daily chores. At the same time, food intakes were less fattening because our forbears did not have the incredible choice of rich ready-made foods in easily accessible shops. There was no question then of having artificially to insert some form of 'activity' into their lives in order to offset any problems caused by a sedentary lifestyle.

The lack of physical fitness of the British population has been recognised as a growing problem throughout this century. The need to set up physical exercise programmes was being discussed by government committees as far back as 1904. The establishment of the Sports Council by the government in 1965 was an indication of how much officialdom recognised the need to persuade all of us to get moving.

These days, for most of us, the physical and manual element has disappeared from our working and home lives and unless we want to grow flabby and unhealthy, we must consciously introduce regular sport or exercise into our lives.

What do you do for a living?

In terms of occupation, the manual working class jobs tend to be more physically demanding than the professional or clerical jobs. On the whole, the more qualified a person is and, generally speaking, the more money they earn, the less likely their job is to offer the degree of personal activity required to keep them in peak physical condition.

The Allied Dunbar National Fitness survey, carried out between 1990 and 1992, was sponsored by The Sports Council, the Health Education Authority and the Department of Health. It also found that nearly half of all men (48%) and 40% of all women are overweight. This shows a dramatic increase compared with a decade earlier when 39% of men and 32% of women were recorded as being overweight.

Strength levels were also measured and it was found that a third of men and half of all women did not have sufficient muscle strength to lift half their bodyweight. As a result, this means that they would, for example, not be able to get up from sitting in a chair without using their arms.

Leg strength was also measured and it was found that over 50% of women aged over 55 had muscles so weak that they would find it increasingly difficult to climb stairs without assistance.

What was particularly interesting about this survey was that there was a huge mismatch about what people thought their state of fitness was and what it actually was. Also, while 80% said they believed in the value of keeping fit, only a tiny minority had actually done anything about it.

Fitness was perceived not only as desirable but also as having been effortlessly attained by four out of five people interviewed. So we have not only a clear case of mass self-deception but also a serious problem of under-recognition of the problem. If you don't even realise that you are unfit, how on earth can you embark on a programme to get into better physical shape?

ARE YOU UNFIT?

This book will give you some simple ways of finding out whether you are part of this majority of unfit adults, as well as suggesting practical ways in which you can bring about improvements.

For health benefits to accrue, whatever form of physical activity you adopt must be maintained. So if your lifestyle involves gardening, walking or cycling – i.e. everyday things that can easily become an integral part of your life – this is much easier to keep going than some form of sport which may decline as other demands impose themselves or an injury occurs.

Even those who currently take part regularly in sport (and probably aren't in need of this book) will have to make lifestyle changes as they get older and when they retire from work in order to maintain their activity levels.

It doesn't have to hurt to get fit so forget 'going for the burn'. If the thought of an exercise bike or a gymnasium has you reaching for the biscuit tin or another bottle of beer, don't worry.

There are other ways in which you can shape up.

- All you are aiming for is finding some ways to incorporate more activity into your everyday life. If you can't stand the thought of vigorous exercise, then the good news is that even moderate-level activity can improve your health. The aim is to try to do some activities for half an hour a day that make your heart beat slightly faster, and leave you feeling a little out of breath. Try to build up so that you are doing this on most days of the week.
- Alternatively, if you do like jogging, fast cycling or other more vigorous exercises, twenty minutes or so continuous exercise just three times a week is enough to improve your level of fitness.

CHAPTER TWO

How fit and active are you?

Most people in Britain think that they are reasonably fit and active. But the question is, fit for what? Our sedentary lives means that a high level of physical fitness dosn't seem necessary, yet we could all benefit from being more physically active.

The most reliable way to assess your fitness accurately is to seek professional help. Private check ups and human MOTs can be expensive though. (If you want more information on professional help, go to p. 16.) Your GP may talk about preventive health and nag you to 'lose weight' or 'stop smoking', but s/he may look aghast if you ask for a complete check-over. So, before you start your new programme of physical activity, try the simple walking test below, and see how you improve as you become fitter.

First though, ask yourself the following questions before starting any new programme of physical activity [*Source* PAR-Q Validation Report, British Columbia Department of Health, June 1975, modified version]:

● Has your doctor ever said you have heart trouble?

● Do you frequently suffer from pains in your chest?

● Do you often feel faint or have spells of severe dizziness?

● Has your doctor ever said your blood pressure was too high?

● Has a doctor ever told you that you have a bone or joint problem such as arthritis that has been aggravated by exercise, or might be made worse by exercise?

● Is there a good reason not mentioned here why you should not follow an activity programme even if you wanted to?

● Are you over age 65 and not accustomed to vigorous exercise?

If the answer is 'yes' to any of these questions, make sure that you consult your GP before embarking on any exercise programme. Your doctor will then be able to check your medical history in greater detail via your medical records.

If you answered 'no' to all of the questions, the following simple walking test will set you on your way to a new active life. Try it!

Walking test

1. Find a safe walking route that takes you about 4–6 minutes to complete. This route doesn't have to be flat or any specific distance.
2. Walk the route. You don't have to walk at any particular speed, but try to walk quite briskly for the full distance of the route.
3. Time how long it takes you to complete the walk, to the nearest second, and take your pulse rate as soon as you have finished.
4. Write down the following:
● the time it took to walk the route
● your pulse rate as soon as you had finished
● how you felt (puffed, tired, ok, etc).

As you become more active and get fitter, you should note some changes, e.g. your walking time may be less, your pulse rate immediately after the walk could drop, or both! And you should be able to complete the walk without feeling so puffed and tired.

Your Get Fitter Programmes

Depending on your current level of activity, try one of the following physical activity programmes:

Get Set! This is for the currently physically inactive. Your aim is to put physical activity into your daily life, gradually building up to being active for 30 minutes on five days or more a week.

Go! is for those who are doing some activity already, but want to feel the benefits of a more structured programme. Your aim is to increase the intensity of your physical activity by having a go at some more vigorous exercises or sports.

For both programmes, six weeks of activity is a good 'activity block'. You may find it easier, too, to be more active, more often, with the help of an 'activity partner' – a friend or relative who also wants to enjoy the benefits of regular physical activity.

Get set!

If you are currently inactive, start gently by choosing ways of doing everyday things that require a little more energy. Listed below are some of the small ways in which you can be more active every day. Choose the ones that suit you

At work:
- use the stairs instead of the lift
- take a brisk walk at lunchtime
- stand up at your desk and stretch every half hour
- imagine that you're late for a meeting and walk a little faster
- dust off that old bike and cycle to work once a week
- park the car further from the office and walk the extra distance
- if you normally go by public transport, try getting off the bus one stop earlier and walking the rest of the way.

At home:
- swap your lawn-mower for a non-motorised one
- stand up and enjoy a stretch during the advert breaks on TV
- dance to one extra record when you go out

- hide the batteries from the TV remote control!
- take the family for a regular swimming session
- plan a regular, brisk, Sunday walk
- walk the dog more often (even if you haven't got a dog!)

Gradually, as you get used to being more active, aim to make your activities last a little longer. It is best if the activity you do is continuous. If possible, it should be demanding enough to make you breathe harder and a little faster, and raise your pulse slightly.

Now that you've got going, you can choose from the following list of moderate intensity activities

- brisk walking (not strolling)
- slow cycling (not getting out of breath)
- stair climbing
- dancing (all kinds)
- slow swimming (not racing)
- digging the garden
- low-impact aerobics
- tennis (doubles)
- jogging/running at a gentle pace.

Don't leap into activities that may be described as 'vigorous' in intensity. These are more demanding and may leave you stiff and sore if you do too much of them, especially if you have been inactive for any length of time. However, within a few weeks even quite vigorous physical activity will feel much easier and pose few problems. But remember – vigorous activity is not necessary in order to improve your physical well – being: it doesn't have to be hell to be healthy!

At the end of six weeks or so of increased physical activity or exercise, try the walking test again, and see how you do now.

Go!

Now's the time to really get going...

Getting fitter

If you are already active, but want to become fitter, more active, and to fully appreciate all the health and fitness benefits of regular physical activity, you will need to increase the amount of time you spend exercising. You may like to increase the intensity of your activity sessions, if appropriate. However, you should never feel dizzy, faint, or desperately breathless; this is a sign that you're over-doing it!

Defining your goals

If you are currently physically active for at least 30 minutes on most days of the week but you would like to do more; you will need to define your goals. In other words, what would you like to see and achieve as a result of your physical activity programme over the next six weeks? Do you want to be generally fitter and in better shape? Are you trying to get fit for a specific sport? Or, are you aiming to lose weight?

Your six week 'activity block' may be used to achieve those goals. The following pointers will help you on your way:

Mixing and matching The most interesting way to become generally fitter is to alternate your activities. This is also a good approach to take if you wish to minimise 'overuse' type injuries.

Mix and match your aerobic activities to involve different muscles in different ways; as long as you exercise at the same relative intensity, you will notice similar improvements in general fitness. For example, you may like to combine running and swimming, or aerobics and cycling, etc. You may like to add 1–2 circuit training, weight training or body conditioning sessions each week to your stamina activities for total fitness benefits. But remember to keep supple by stretching thoroughly as part of your warm-up and cool-down phases.

Getting fit for sport Use your six-week activity block to improve your general conditioning, whatever your sport. Improve your general stamina or endurance through steady pace aerobic activity (running, cycling, swimming, rowing, etc – whichever is most appropriate) lasting at least 20 minutes according to your fitness level, 2–3 times per week. You could also try some general circuit training, weight training, or high repetition weight training, 2–3 times per week (sports or leisure centre staff should be able to advise).

Remember to stretch comprehensively as part of your warm-up and cool-down. Such preparatory training will allow you to move easily into speed and strength training with a much reduced risk of injury.

Losing weight One of the major advantages of regular physical activity is that it can help everyone lose weight and maintain their correct weight level. This is in stark contrast to a 'diet' where it is not unusual for a person's weight to 'yo-yo' between light and heavy.

Aerobic exercise (which uses fat as fuel) is recommended, especially if it is continuous and lasts upwards of 30 minutes per session, 3–5 times weekly. But specific strengthening exercises such as weight training, circuit training, body conditioning, etc, are also useful since these tone and condition muscles at the same time. And, if you increase the amount of muscle you have, you will burn more calories, since muscle uses up energy even at rest.

Combined with sensible eating habits, such an exercise programme is certain to lead to improved shape and fat loss. Furthermore, your activity will ensure that the fat stays off!

After six weeks or so of increased physical activity or exercise, try the walking test once again, and see how you do now.

PROFESSIONAL HELP

Prior to starting any physical activity programme, you may prefer to get some expert help in assessing how fit you are. There is no shortage of options. The main ones are

● your GP (especially if you are elderly)
● private health insurance companies – e.g. BUPA or PPP
● sports/health clubs.

YOUR GP

Unfortunately, unless you are very lucky, your GP won't be able to help much, beyond agreeing that it would be a good idea to get fit and endorsing your plans. Although a few enlightened GPs around the country are beginning to prescribe a fitness programme for some of their patients – particularly those suffering from depression – most are not clued up in this respect.

However, what your GP can do is help you to look at your general state of health. S/he can and should take your blood pressure on a fairly regular basis, and s/he should be able to pass comment on your weight as it relates to your health. Consulting your GP is well worth doing as s/he will have access to your medical records and can advise you specifically rather than generally, as this book can merely do.

PRIVATE HEALTH

You can have virtually anything tested if you are prepared to pay for the privilege. An increasing number of companies are offering their employees free or heavily subsidised health screening services. It is just as much in their interests to have a healthy workforce as it is in yours to ensure that you keep in peak physical shape.

Whether you have encountered any health problems or not – maybe a back injury, or you have had rather too many headaches and taken a lot of time off from work lately – a thorough fitness check-up may be worth while.

All the big private health companies offer full screening services for men and women. If you are thinking of this, look out in the newspapers and magazines for any 'special offers', as quite good deals come up from time to time. Shop around as prices do vary.

A full private check-up with any of the big companies costs anything from £150 to £350, partly depending on how many tests they carry out. Your company may operate a discount scheme – so do ask. Or there may be discounts for groups of, say, six people, so it might be worth getting together with some other people.

These hospitals are expensive to run. They therefore need to keep finding new patients and so, even if you think it might turn out to be too expensive, it's probably worth making a few phone calls and inquiring. With a bit of luck, a special deal may be made. If not, consider the investment in yourself. After all, when you compare the cost of a health screen to the amount you spend on clothes and hairdressing appointments, it is not such a big price to pay.

SPORTS/HEALTH CLUBS

If you are interested mainly in physical fitness and are not worried about your general health, a sports club might be the best place for you. Private health clubs automatically offer their members full fitness testing and there is no limit usually on the number of assessments you can have.

The advantage of a private fitness assessment by someone professionally qualified is that they will be able to take account of your lifestyle and attitude as well as your general level of fitness before prescribing a programme that is tailor-made for you.

You may, for example, say that you are not going to be able to get to the gym more than once a week and that you find it hard to get motivated, in which case your assessor will probably suggest a suitable class for your level of fitness to enable you to keep to a timetable.

An experienced instructor will know that, once you get into the habit of calling in at the health club for a weekly class, it is but a small step to come in a second time for a workout in the gym and, who knows, maybe for a second class?

The main advantage of an individual fitness assessment is that whoever you consult will be able to look into any past injuries or ill-health and test each aspect of your overall fitness as well as doing basic testing on your heart rate, blood pressure, fat percentages, and so on.

Modern clubs have computerised programmes that allow the assessors to feed in your initial test results and give you a print-out. It is a good idea to pin these up on your fridge door, where they will dissuade you from going berserk when you are starving!

These print-outs should be kept as you can then compare how you do at subsequent assessments. If you have made good progress, they can be very encouraging.

Your assessor may find surprising things, such as that you have very strong arms, or even one strong arm, but very weak calves, or very flexible hips but stiff shoulders. Whatever s/he finds, a specific exercise will be available to work on that part of the body in order to improve your overall fitness levels.

Private health clubs can be very expensive, but most local authority-run sports and leisure centres offer similar services, albeit in somewhat less-luxurious settings. Most run short, once-a-week courses you can go to after work in specific activities, from basketball to yoga, or just plain exercise classes. Even if you don't know where your nearest centre is, you should make a point of looking it up and you may be surprised at the range of what's on offer ... and how cheap some of the courses can be.

Don't just look near where you live. There may be a good leisure centre near your work, or on the way between home and work, which may be just as convenient.

CHAPTER THREE

Why be fit?

Think about why exactly it is that you want to become fit. You will probably say that you want to be slimmer, you want your body to be firm and toned, and you have heard that a fit body is less likely to succumb to disease.

That's all true, but the benefits of becoming fit are not only physical, they are also psychological.

THE PSYCHOLOGICAL BENEFITS OF FITNESS

Becoming fit is not merely a physical act, fitness is also a state of mind. You will find it easier and more enjoyable to achieve your chosen state of fitness if you have 'psyched' yourself into it.

Rather like people's attitude to giving up smoking (you have to really want to give up in order to succeed), you also need to really want to get fit in order to do it. It helps to have a motive or target.

Motivating yourself

For those who have been fit before, and can remember how good and positive they felt, recalling those more energetic days may be quite enough in itself to inspire them to get back into shape. Maybe they were a mini-star in the school football or hockey team, or they managed to win a cup in a swimming contest at college, or perhaps they won the darts championship down at the local pub before they moved house and started a family.

For them, resuming an old sport or activity will be easier because they may still have some contacts and at least know where to look for the nearest swimming pool, riding stables, badminton team, or whatever.

For those whose present state of unfitness has been a general downhill slide since they can't remember when, recalling past glories, never mind looking up old team-mates, may not be possible.

For them, the motivation might be a holiday coming up where they want to be able to do more than lie on the beach, semi-covered up, envying those of a more athletic and graceful appearance. Or it could be a big birthday – 40 is often a time when people look at their horrible middle-aged bulges and wonder if it might *not* be inevitable that they get larger and rounder with each passing year.

It might simply be that you are finding yourself in a constant state of lethargy. 'Can't be bothered' is becoming your automatic reaction to every suggestion of what you might do – whether for work or pleasure – and you want to snap out of it.

Once you have pinpointed your motive, perhaps you should write it down, or write a letter to a good friend stating your aim, or declare your intentions to your loved ones. In this way, it keeps the motive 'alive'. The people you've chosen to confide in will ask for regular updates – which is in itself an incentive not to give up!

Stress

Maybe you are feeling stressed at work and finding that life is all a bit too frenetic. The result is that you're feeling wound up most of the time.

Stress is bad for us and, unchecked, it can lead not only to physical but also mental illness. Stress is a sense of frustration which turns frequently to anger. It is that powerful feeling of frustration and anger which we feel when we are held up in a traffic jam. Sometimes we react by doing silly things like driving much too fast when we are free of the jam, or by jumping out of the car and threatening violence to anyone who gets in the way.

We all have in-built stress levels, which, to a certain extent, are essential to our well-being. The so-called 'fight-or-flight' response is necessary for those times when we are put under severe stress and need to be able to react with our maximum potential. Adrenalin is a hormone which is released at such times, causing the pulse rate and blood pressure to rise, our muscles to tense and our glands to sweat.

Unfortunately, because the physical energy required to get most of us through our daily lives is now so very low, the adrenalin we have stored in our bodies ready for such 'fight-or-flight' responses gets used whenever we feel tense, frightened, angry or excited. This then spills over, causing many other problems – insomnia, headaches, and an inability to concentrate, perhaps underlined by a general feeling that you are just not coping with life.

Dealing with stress

There are two main ways of dealing with stress. The first is relaxation, and the second is exercise.

Relaxation comes more easily to some people than to others. The easiest way to relax is to sit back, play some soothing music and just forget about the world and its worries.

It sounds simple but some of us find it surprisingly hard to do. No matter how hard we try to empty our heads of worries, they soon start creeping back into our minds, and our so-called relaxation session has left us no better off – maybe even worse than before because we've now 'wasted' our all-too-precious time.

You can also try relaxing through finding time in your day to lie down and do some deep breathing exercises or meditate.

Exercise is one of the best ways of relieving stress and tension. Exercise is known to release certain natural chemicals in the brain, which make you feel happy and relaxed. The sense of well-being and relaxation that you experience after exercising lasts for much longer than the period during which you are actually being active.

Even a short walk clears the head and makes you feel better but this is only a short-term solution. Regular exercise fitted into your weekly schedules will ensure that the stress build-up simply doesn't occur.

How not to deal with stress

However tempting, try not to resort to 'quick fixes' to alleviate stress. Most of these are very deceptive – although they may initially offer comfort, they are all unhealthy and may eventually lead to illness.

- **Don't have a stiff drink.**
- **Don't smoke.**
- **Don't hit the biscuit-tin.**
- **Don't drink lots of cups of coffee – caffeine is a stimulant and only increases tension.**
- **Don't resort to tranquillisers for anything but a short-term crisis.**
- **Don't give up on exercise.**

Exercise makes you feel better

Exercise is definitely good for lifting the spirits – that is official! It is confirmed by a number of research studies in different parts of the world, particularly in European countries and the USA.

An increasing number of GPs have realised the connection between being unfit and depression. In some cases, they have begun prescribing a fitness programme rather than doling out yet more anti-depressants.

The link between exercise and stress has been studied by Professor Steptoe and his colleagues at the Psychology Department of St George's Medical School in London. They have found that adults in a normal state of health, benefit from exercise. Volunteers were asked to do 20 minutes of vigorous exercise three or four times a week. These people were compared to others who merely undertook light exercising during the same 10-week period. Anxiety, tension and depression levels were all measured both before and after the programme.

All those taking part in the programme, whatever the level of exercising they had been allocated, found that tension, depression and anxiety levels were reduced. But those who were exercising hardest experienced much greater reductions and they all found that they could cope better with whatever stresses they encountered in their daily lives.

A recent study in Norway went even further than this. It showed that psychiatric patients who were already hospitalised by their severe state of mental illness showed considerable improvement in psychological well-being when persuaded to do an hour's steady jogging three times week. It took most of the patients between six to nine weeks to get fully fit, working at between 50–70% of their maximum aerobic capacity. Most were normally fit by the time they were discharged. All of them were given their usual medication and other therapy such as counselling but by the end of the experiment, those who had been exercising regularly were substantially less depressed than the non-exercising in-patients.

It was also found that when the exercising patients were offered a choice of aerobic exercise (jogging) or non-aerobic exercise (weight-lifting), there was no particular difference in the outcome, suggesting that *any* form of regular exercise was better than none.

The doctors found that all the patients who had become mentally ill were seriously unfit (and this finding has been noticed elsewhere). This is not to say that if you become unfit you will automatically end up in a mental hospital but it does suggest that if you have suffered from depression in the past, or are perhaps going through a low phase right now, under-activity could be an important factor.

What has not yet been shown is whether sedentary and less fit people become depressed because they are sedentary and unfit, or whether people become less active and unfit because they are depressed. It would be fascinating to find out.

THE PHYSICAL BENEFITS OF EXERCISE

Overall, your body will be effectively 'younger' and healthier than the bodies of your non-exercising friends and colleagues. Specifically, there are 12 major benefits that you can expect to enjoy once you have improved your all-round fitness by following the ideas in this book.

- You will sleep more soundly than before.
- You will wake up feeling more energetic.
- Your muscles and joints will stay in efficient working order as long as you maintain your fitness levels.
- You will strengthen your bones so there is less risk of bone-thinning (osteoporosis) and a reduced risk of fractures should you fall.
- You will improve your circulation so that blood reaches all parts of your body more efficiently.
- You may well lose weight and maintain your ideal weight levels.
- Your body will be in better shape and look more attractive, in and out of clothes, as muscles replace fat.
- The proportion of fat in your body may decrease.
- Your blood pressure will be lowered if it's prone to being on the high side, while if it's normal, it will stay normal.
- Your heart will become stronger so that it can do its normal

workload more easily and have a bigger reserve capacity.
- Stress levels may be reduced. If you suffer from stress-related symptoms such as headaches, migraines or indigestion, these may subside.
- You may reduce the cholesterol levels in your blood, reducing fatty deposits in your arteries and thus preventing the build-up, which, if unchecked, leads to strokes and heart attacks.

Are you convinced?

Does this all sound too good to be true? Are you secretly convinced that this exercise fad is just a 'con'?

Fortunately, in the last few decades, an immense amount of research has been carried out into the merits of exercise and each and every one of the statements above can be verified. But for these claims to have any significance, it is not merely a question of hopping on an exercise bike three times a week and assuming that all will be well. After all, it is no good being fit as a fiddle if you lead an otherwise unhealthy lifestyle.

Even the fittest can drop dead from a heart attack and even the fleetest of foot can be killed in a car accident or sustain serious permanent injury in some kind of disaster. But, generally speaking, by getting fitter and improving your overall health, you should increase the odds of staying well and staying alive – for longer.

CHAPTER FOUR

Heart disease

Heart disease is Britain's most common form of death. Could you die from it?

How unhealthy is your lifestyle, given that most of us lead lives that are much too inactive for our own good? Technological developments have given us a wealth of labour-saving devices. While making life easier, these also progressively make us less healthy.

LIVING A LIFE OF LUXURY

From the minute you get out of bed in the morning, life is easy. You emerge from your bed to a warm, centrally heated home (no energy expended warming up your chilled body), you throw the duvet back on the bed (no 10-minute stretch as you make the bed). You step into the shower or bath, full of hot-running water (no boiler-stoking to get the warmth into the house).

Then it's downstairs for a quick slice of ready-sliced toast in the toaster (no slicing, no sharpening of the knife, no cooking dexterity required). You'll probably have some instant coffee, and you'll put some instant washing-up in the dishwasher. Then you'll go out to the car, off to work, park the car, into the office-building, up the lift, on to the phone, sit at your 'work-station' all day. Maybe the most energetic demand you make of your body is changing gear in the car and making that trip to the coffee-machine?

Meanwhile, back home, you pop a ready-made meal into the microwave, then pop your feet up to spend an average of 25 hours a week watching TV and the video. The remote control means you don't even have to cross the room to change channel.

Still we seek yet more labour-saving devices until, eventually, we will hardly have to stir out of bed to go shopping. More and more restaurants deliver food to our door. With the rapid increase in home-working, many of us won't even have to step outside the warmth of our homes to earn a living.

The dangers of under-activity

Under-activity is unhealthy and can lead to serious disease and even premature death. Whether you are male or female, heart disease is the number one killer. About half of all deaths in the UK are caused by either coronary or artery diseases of the heart.

A definite association has now been made between the high incidence of coronary heart disease and low levels of physical activity. The converse is also true. Research confirms that the risk is inversely related to the time spent being physically active.

How much physical activity is enough?

For maximum health benefits, physical activity has to be regular. Activity at a moderate level, such as brisk walking (about 3–4mph) burns off about 5 kcal a minute, and should leave you feeling slightly warm and out of breath. If this is the level of activity that you enjoy, the aim should be to build up to around 30 minutes of this type of activity on five or more days of the week.

Vigorous activities, such as jogging or running, need to be done less often to improve fitness levels. Activities like these expend around 7.5 kcal per minute, and usually would leave you feeling pretty puffed afterwards. They should be maintained for at least 20 minutes and done at least three times a week. If the metabolic rate is 'charged' in this way on a regular basis, the heart pumps at its best and the long-term risk of suffering a heart attack can be reduced by 50%.

Various studies have demonstrated that lack of physical activity contributes to the risk of coronary heart disease as much as hypertension (high blood pressure). If you have more than one of these risk factors – i.e. you have high blood pressure and/or still smoke, as well as lead a sedentary lifestyle – your chances of making it to a ripe old age are more remote.

Does this sound like you – and most of your colleagues? This may sound depressing, but the good news is that it's never too late to start getting fitter – however out of condition your body has become and however hopeless a case you might feel.

Most people reach their peak physical strength in their early 20s but, according to Ian Chaffey, Fitness Manager at the Mecklenburgh Health Club in London, this can be maintained well into your 40s and 50s as long as you keep working your body all the time.

Trouble arises, though, if you don't do this. 'Both muscle-power and cardiovascular fitness slip away at the frightening rate of 10% a decade if we maintain just a minimum level of activity,' he says.

The only way to make up for this natural decline is through regular physical activity, and if neither your job nor your home-life offers scope for this, then you have to find some-thing active to put into your lifestyle. Fortunately, the body's response to exercise is very rewarding, and the physical effects are surprisingly swift, reversing the damage wrought by years of inactivity and bad habits like smoking and drinking.

HIGH BLOOD PRESSURE

It's all very well for you lot, you might say, but what about those of us who've got high blood pressure anyway? We're already doomed – so what's the point of keeping fit?

Well, the point is that by exercising regularly, you can in fact permanently lower your blood pressure. Research has shown that moderate intense rhythmic exercise can lower blood pressure to below the danger levels of 140/90mm Hg.

High blood pressure can of course be treated with drugs. But as these will have to be taken for the rest of your life, how much better to keep active and perhaps do without pills, especially as no medicines come without undesirable side-effects?

About 10–15% of the adult population suffer from high blood pressure and we know from all the evidence that these people are three times more likely to have a heart attack, and four times more likely to have heart failure, than those whose blood pressure is normal.

A heart attack in someone who is hypertensive is more likely to be fatal than in someone whose blood pressure is normal. If you have high blood pressure and you smoke, your risk of having a stroke is 12 times that of those leading healthier lives, and if you drink alcohol in large quantities, the risk is aggravated still further.

As Dr David Ashton, Clinical Director of BMI Healthcare and The London Heart Clinic, notes in his book *The 12 Week Executive Health Plan*: 'Small wonder that insurance companies take careful note of an individual's blood pressure when determining life insurance premiums.'

It has been demonstrated that in as little as eight weeks, a programme of vigorous exercise can dramatically reduce blood pressure and also improve the circulation. Age is no barrier – within months, fit men and women in their 40s and 50s can outperform unfit people in their 20s and 30s.

Only a male problem?

According to the latest report from the British Family Heart Study, published in February 1994, nearly one in five men has high blood pressure and only marginally fewer women. The study, which is based on nearly 4,000 patients from all over the country, noted that the risk of heart disease is hardly any lower in women compared with men.

It says: 'Cardiovascular disease is still the commonest cause of premature death among women.' As women compete with men at work, at all levels, their patterns of disease become similar to men's and so they must take similar precautions to avoid heart disease in all its forms.

The researchers noted that it was crucial to include women not only in their own right, but because 'women still hold the main responsibility for shopping and cooking. They are therefore in a powerful position to influence the dietary habits of the whole family.'

It is true that women's hormones offer some protection against coronary heart disease, but after the menopause their risks catch up with the men's. But it is also true that women who develop heart disease are twice as likely to die from a first attack as men are, and if they survive, they are twice as likely to have a second attack.

The image still lingers in most people's minds that it is the stressed-out, middle-aged, high-flying executive who gets heart disease. This was certainly the case up to 30 or 40 years ago, but things have changed and it is now primarily the unskilled and manual workers. There are exceptions, but as a general rule, the higher up the work and social ladder you go, the lower your risks of dying of coronary heart disease.

What we don't know for sure, but can only make intelligent guesses about, is that the reduced risk has something to do with the fact that smoking habits follow a similar pattern – as do exercise patterns.

CORONARY HEART DISEASE

Most people recognise that coronary heart disease is dangerous and the vast majority of us presume that it has always been so. But this is definitely not the case. It is very much a disease of our times. Before the last World War, doctors rarely treated anyone for the disease and deaths from it were almost as rare as deaths from measles today.

Cholesterol levels among the general population are so high that two-thirds of us ought to be doing something to lower them, mainly through altering our diet and increasing our exercise levels. As well as the better-known risks of high cholesterol levels in the blood, newer research shows that fibrinogen, a special protein which aids blood clotting, also plays a crucial role, possibly equal to that of high cholesterol, in predicting the chances of heart disease.

Moderate rhythmic exercise increases fibrinolytic activity and reduces platelet aggregation of the blood, which prevents clots forming. Clots are what cause thrombosis – the condition that sees off so many middle-aged men well before their allotted three score and ten (or 20 if they are lucky!).

Facts and figures

● One in three men and one in four women will die from it.
● Thanks to coronary heart disease, 27,000 men never make it to 65 years old and miss out on their retirement altogether.
● In 1991, 170,000 people in the UK died from the disease. This was made up of 92,000 men and 78,000 women.
● The UK, including Scotland and Ireland, tops the world for deaths from heart disease.

Running in the family?

Certain families are definitely more prone to some diseases than others and heart disease is no exception – indeed, it is the prime example.

It is the case that heart disease tends to run in families but scientists do not yet know whether this is something that comes from the genes or whether families tend to replicate the bad habits – like poor diet or smoking – that they have grown up with.

Whatever the reason, if you have a close relative – say, a mother, father, brother or sister – who died prematurely from heart disease while under the age of 60, this is counted as a definite risk factor for YOU.

This does not mean that you WILL die from heart disease, merely that you need to be extra careful to make sure that the dice are not loaded against you in other ways. You cannot do anything to alter your genes, but you can modify all the other factors that could make your future health prospects look more appetising!

In some cases high cholesterol levels run in the family. This condition is called familial hypercholesterolaemia (FH) and is linked with increased risk of premature heart disease (under 55 years of age in women and under 50 years of age in men). However, it can be treated with dietary change and/or drugs.

The main risk factors are
- **Smoking**
- **High blood pressure**
- **Physical inactivity**
- **Raised blood cholesterol**
- **Obesity**

MAKING YOUR HEART FITTER

Can you climb a flight of 20 stairs without getting breathless? According to fitness experts, you should be able to do that at the age of 45. You should also be able to run a mile in 10 minutes and your resting heartbeat should be about 65 beats per minute.

If you are younger than this and you know you can't accomplish any stairs without getting breathless, you don't need me to tell you you are unfit. You probably just haven't stopped to think about it before, because becoming unfit is a progressive event. You don't usually notice it happening.

Just like a car which pumps petrol as soon as you start the engine and press on the accelerator, so as you start to exercise, your heart literally needs to pump more blood round your body. Fitness training simply improves your heart's performance – rather like having your engine tuned would improve your car's.

There, though, the analogy stops. Measuring how well your heart is performing is not quite as easy as listening to how sweetly a well-tuned engine runs.

The easiest way to measure (and monitor the improvement in) your heart's functioning is to measure your resting pulse rate. The typical non-smoker has an average pulse rate of between 65 to 70 beats a minute. Smokers' pulses beat between 70-80 beats a minute.

In general, the lower your pulse rate is, the more efficiently your heart is working so that once you have increased your fitness levels, your resting pulse rate should fall to 60 beats per minute, or even lower.

However, it is not only the resting pulse that we are interested in. After exercise, the pulse rate quickens, but this speeds up vastly more among those who are unfit than among those who are fit. After a bout of vigorous exercise, say running for a bus, a fit person will have a pulse rate of say 80 or 90 beats a minute whereas an unfit person may have a pulse rate of 120 or even more.

Cardiac output

The human body contains around 11 pints of blood, which have to be pumped around all parts of the body constantly. The amount of blood the heart pumps in a minute is called its cardiac output.

At rest, the heart pumps all 11 pints in about a minute – a remarkable feat if you stop to think about it, especially as it does this 24 hours a day, seven days a week. During an average lifetime, a heart will beat an awesome three billion times. Do you know any other machine that works so efficiently?

A fit heart beats less often per minute than an unfit one and so the amount of blood it pumps at each stroke – the stroke rate – is greater. The heart's stroke volume increases substantially with vigorous exercise. When extra demands are placed upon it – like running for the bus or running up the stairs, the heart of an unfit person has to beat much faster than the heart of a fit person which merely pumps more blood with each stroke.

Thrombosis

The truly remarkable thing about the heart is that this stupendous organ is supplied with all its vital fuel – the blood – through two tiny arteries, about an eighth of an inch in diameter. It is these tiny coronary arteries that are, literally, our lifeline.

They can become blocked with fatty deposits, or plaque. If the build-up goes on unchecked, it can result in the artery blocking completely, resulting in a thrombosis or blood clot. If this happens, the blood, which carries oxygen to every part of the body, including the brain and heart, ceases to flow. Since these can only survive without oxygen for a couple of minutes or so, unless emergency supplies are provided, the result will be a heart attack as far as the heart is concerned, or a stroke as far as the brain is concerned. Either way, sudden death can be the outcome.

Angina

Luckily for some people, they get a clear warning. This is known as angina, a condition where the arteries have thickened and the heart is starved periodically of oxygen.

This usually manifests itself during a period of exercise when, as the heart-rate increases, so does the demand for oxygen. The partially blocked arteries cannot deliver the amount of oxygen required by the heart and so the person concerned suffers a gripping painful sensation across the chest. Some people feel as though something is crushing them in the chest while others feel as if they are being strangled round their throats. Others may have pains in their arms, particularly their left arms, while some may merely get a sensation of pins and needles in their fingers. All of these are possible as a result of vigorous activity and the pain subsides once the person has rested.

It is estimated that between 2–3 million people suffer from angina in the UK and most take drugs to control their condition, while some have to undergo surgery. It is a foolish person who ignores this kind of pain when they have been forced to exert themselves, e.g. running for a bus or walking up a steepish hill.

Stroke

When the arteries to the brain become blocked, the brain is starved of oxygen and a stroke will result.

A stroke can either kill you instantly, or it can leave some form of permanent or semi-permanent disability or one or other side of the body.

Although death through strokes is rightly seen as a disease affecting mainly the elderly, it is by no means exclusive to the aged. For while strokes do mainly affect the elderly, about 25,000 people aged under 65 have one each year, of whom nearly 5,000 drop dead instantly.

CHAPTER FIVE

Choosing the right exercise for you

It is impossible to say which is the best physical activity for you. Only you can decide that, depending on your age, your personality, your routine, your lifestyle – in other words, everything about you.

Start with the exercise that is most accessible, and most pleasing, to you. The following activities are all highly recommended.

WALKING

The great thing about walking is that you start at your own pace, quite literally. Because it is not weight-bearing or competitive, you are unlikely to suffer any worse injuries than the odd blister!

Psychologically, walking is a very good way of relieving stress and tension. There's nothing like a good walk to get rid of some pent-up anger or frustration.

It is safe and can be done virtually anywhere, any time, alone or in company. You can do it with friends or with the dog.

Maybe you can walk to work, or do it in your lunch hour. Why not invite a colleague or two to go with you? You could even talk over important business matters while out walking, rather than doing it in a smoky stuffy atmosphere. You may find you can all think more clearly – and you'll certainly feel fresher when the 'meeting' is over!

Walking for fitness means that you should aim to work up a bit of a sweat and get out of breath. So this excludes the gentlest of ambles round the park, or window shopping round all your favourite haunts.

After building up gradually, you should be able to walk briskly for half an hour without being so exhausted that you can't even hold a conversation – even if you are puffing somewhat. Hills are useful to build up muscles in your legs and to work your heart muscles even harder.

Ordinary flat comfortable shoes are fine but if you get the 'bug', it is worth investing in a properly designed pair of walking shoes.

JOGGING AND RUNNING

These are merely faster and more strenuous versions of walking and the same guidelines apply. However, because you are moving faster, your feet will hit the ground harder and may jar your joints and muscles so you could strain yourself, especially your knees, hips, ankles and feet.

If you have arthritis or if you are overweight, swimming or cycling are safer bets. Don't run or jog so fast that you wear yourself out in five minutes flat, as the length of time you spend doing this kind of aerobic exercise is much more important than the speed you can get up to! Try to keep to soft surfaces like grass and invest in a good pair of running shoes. If you're not lucky enough to be by the sea or in the country, try and exercise in parks rather than along busy roads.

INDOOR CYCLING/ROWING MACHINES

Unlike most forms of exercise, these do not rely on the weather being favourable as you can put the machine in any room in your house – or even in a corner at work! Having it in front of the TV is more likely to keep you exercising as without music or the radio or some other distraction, this form of exercise can be dull.

If you're not sure how much time you can spare for exercise, a machine might be ideal. A stationary machine is good if you are overweight because you can't over-balance.

Keep your back straight while you cycle or row and make sure that you rotate your muscles fully, but never overdo it. A meter which measures how 'far' you've been is useful so that you can increase your 'mileage' each day. Adjustments which make it easier and harder to pedal will vary the pace and help you to get fitter.

If you have a bad back, a rowing machine is not recommended.

SWIMMING

This is the best all-round exercise for everyone because you can use practically every muscle and joint in your body without putting any weight on any of them. You can be pregnant or overweight, elderly and/or arthritic or suffering from backache or even severely handicapped, and still be able to derive a lot of pleasure and health benefits from this excellent form of exercise.

If you can't swim, find out about lessons as it is never too late to learn. Provided you have a nearby pool, it is also very cheap as all you need is a bathing costume and a towel! You may find it is more convenient to swim in a pool near where you work than in one near where you live. A lunch hour swim can be very invigorating.

To swim for aerobic fitness you should swim lengths of breast or backstroke or crawl, building up your stamina until you can swim without stopping to get your breath back for at least 20 minutes.

Once you can swim, a whole range of water-based sports are open to you, from the very athletic surfing, windsurfing and diving to the slightly more leisurely sailing and rowing.

CYCLING

Cycling is a great way to get about, provided you have good road sense and you don't have to be that fit to start with. However, you must have a good natural sense of balance, so practice on a borrowed bike if you are thinking of taking it up for the first time in middle-age.

You may be able to cycle to work, saving you fares and time. Cycling with a purpose – i.e. getting from A to B, rather than merely for activity – confers a sense of freedom and independence which most people find both invigorating and uplifting. You arrive at work (on time!), warmed up and raring to go, rather than raddled and irritated by delays and difficulties experienced by most commuters using other forms of transport.

Cycling for fitness means getting up a good steady (not reckless!) speed for journeys of not less than about 20 minutes, which means that in country areas you should be able to cover as much as 10 miles at a time, and in cities a little less, because of traffic lights, traffic jams and so on.

Wear brightly coloured clothing and good strong shoes. If you are cycling in the city you may decide to wear a mask to reduce the amount of exhaust fumes you inhale from passing traffic. Also, invest in a comfortable good quality helmet. Cyclists are obviously at risk from injury and the head is the most vulnerable part of the body as far as fatal accidents are concerned.

Think about your bike's security as well as your own. You'll also need a strong lock for when you want to stop for a rest and park the bike.

TEAM SPORTS

Ask around at work to see if there is anyone who fancies a game of tennis on a local court. Courts can be found even in the middle of the busiest and most built-up cities so there is no excuse!

Sports like tennis and badminton require not only fitness and stamina but, because they are competitive, they may also expose you to the risk of injury – in stretching for an awkward shot, for example. As such, if you have an existing condition like a bad back, it would be necessary to take expert advice. One particular hazard is 'tennis elbow', which is basically the result of badly executed overarm shots. Poor posture and incorrect technique are often to blame for this condition, so it is worth seeking out a coach for some lessons in correct grip and positioning.

Another possibility is to arrange a five-a-side football team. This is not usually difficult to organise in any company of modest size – suggest one if there isn't one already.

Alternatively, you may prefer a game with friends or neighbours away from work in the local park. But before signing on for your local team, you should put in a few practice sessions and remember to warm up before any proper games or you'll pay the price later in the form of stiff muscles or much worse! In terms of getting fit, it is the training sessions between matches that are probably of more use to you physically then the games themselves.

GOLF

Golf is perhaps the number one game associated with the executive lifestyle. Many is the businessman who swears all his best deals are done on the golf-course.

Combining sport with work seems to be a brilliant idea. If your work lends itself to it, you should definitely kit yourself out with a set of clubs or get down to your nearest golf range as soon as possible.

Golf appears to be a leisurely game, yet is actually quite demanding. You need a high degree of motor-coordination and a lot of strength in your back, shoulders, arms and wrists, plus stamina to walk the several miles of an 18 hole course, pulling a heavy trolley full of clubs.

Experts disagree on how wise it is for people with a pre-existing condition like a weak back to take up golf. As it is a one-sided sport because of the 'swing', and because it also requires you to carry a heavy set of clubs for some distance, it may be unsuitable for some.

If golf appeals, perhaps try putting on its own and then pitch and putting before getting on to a proper golf-course. It may even be a good idea to book a lesson with a pro to see if you are in suitable shape.

SQUASH

Squash is a very fast and demanding game which, even if you play with a 'slow' ball, will exhaust anyone who is not already fairly fit. Squash is not a game in which to try and score points with a business rival or boss – not unless you are very fit indeed and an experienced player!

Try to start playing with a partner who is at a similar standard and level of fitness as yourself so that you don't push yourself too hard. Chasing after the ball in a small enclosed court with hard walls is a very good way of injuring yourself if you don't know how to put the brakes on!

Playing with a partner who is much faster on their feet and fitter than you are can be demoralising and frustrating. If one of you inches ahead, the other either needs to put in some extra training or to find a slower partner.

If you are up to it, squash is an excellent sport for stamina. Being indoors, you are unlikely to breathe anything other than rather hot smelly air so it is certainly unwise for asthmatics or people who have chest problems.

AEROBICS

Just as slimming clubs inspire mutual confidence, an exercise class will keep you at it when solitary activities like walking or swimming might easily be dropped for lack of time, or boredom.

The important thing about an aerobics class is to find a teacher who knows what he or she is doing, to know your own limitations and to book into a class at the appropriate level. If you are a beginner, don't be overambitious. Start in the beginners' class, and even then, drop out when you start to feel tired. Don't try to keep up until you are uncomfortably out of breath.

Many people have injured themselves, some permanently, by pushing themselves too hard in classes which are too fast and advanced for them. Most osteopaths and orthopaedic surgeons have cases involving wrenched muscles, twisted or broken ankles, torn ligaments, slipped discs and all manner of back problems, often incurred during such classes. And there are other health risks – one little-known hazard is vertigo (dizziness) and hearing loss along with tinnitus (the persistent ringing in the ears) which many aerobics teachers have developed after long exposure to loud pounding music along with high-impact exercises.

Some seemingly ordinary exercises like straight sit-ups or push-ups can lead to severe strains and injuries, especially if you do too many in one go. Joints can lock and the lower spine can be compressed. If anything is out of place to start with, vigorous unskilled overuse of any or all parts of the body is going to be risky.

CHAPTER SIX

Avoiding – and dealing with – injury

The reason why you are reading this book is presumably because you want to get into better shape. You are leading a busy life and everything you do has to be carefully fitted into a fairly tough schedule.

The last thing you need is to injure yourself, especially in the course of trying to get fitter! Unfortunately, however, few of us reach middle-age without sustaining some sort of back or joint injury, which not only prevents us getting and staying fit, but can make even basic day-to-day living very difficult.

Many people do their backs in merely by lifting objects awkwardly at work or at home, or by sitting badly at a desk or workbench or in a car, or by spending too much time on their feet. Many a back has been put out by leaping for a bus or a taxi when in too much of a hurry.

Injuries of any kind are going to mean a lot of discomfort. But, more than that, they are also going to mean valuable days lost from work and considerable inconvenience and expense all round.

EXERCISING SAFELY

Think of your body as a relatively high-powered car that spends most of its life doing either nothing at all or short 'stop-start' shopping trips. How good it feels to take it on to an open motorway where you can put your foot down and 'clear the tubes'. Continue with the metaphor though and you will see why too much, too soon, can be potentially dangerous, if not fatal. If you haven't checked the condition of the tyres and kept the car's engine and vital parts in good condition, they may have become clogged (just like your ageing arteries) so that when you put your foot hard down on the accelerator for too long, something snaps and catastrophe occurs.

Most of us who work lead stressful lives – with too much mental activity and not enough physical activity and the result is an imbalance. Whatever form of medicine you believe in – Eastern or Western, one common underlying belief is that most illnesses are caused by physical imbalances.

To avoid injuries and catastrophes, there are five 'golden rules' to remember at all times. As far as exercising itself is concerned, injuries are obviously something of an occupational hazard but, if you take care, barring any dramatic accidents, you can minimise your chances of sustaining a serious injury.

Golden rules

The five golden rules are as follows:

1. **Think long term and get fit gradually – take stairs not lifts and walk whenever you can.**

2. **Warm up before you start playing or exercising as this will lessen the chances of sprains and strains. Have a few gentle bends and stretches and arm-swings.**

3. **Exercise regularly – three 20 minute sessions a week are the best to keep fit – plan them and fit them into your schedule so there's no excuse to drop them.**

4. **Cool down afterwards by walking slowly for a few minutes. If possible have a nice warm bath to relax muscles and joints.**

5. **Keep at it - fitness is ongoing – you can't bottle and store it!**

The warm-up

Perhaps the most important of the golden rules is the warm-up, which you should do before engaging in any form of exercise in order to loosen everything up first.

You've probably seen Mr Motivator and, before him, the Green Goddess on the television doing their five-minute warm-up sessions. The object is just to let your muscles know that they are going to need to work harder than they do normally. If you go straight into tough exercises when your muscles are cold, you are risking injury by over-stretching them.

Expert physiologists will argue over which type of warm-up exercises are best but 'shaking out' is a good basic, as is some running on the spot and bending at the waist and then twisting your trunk. Circling the shoulders forwards and backwards is good, too, as is rotating your head gently, and flexing your knees and balancing on one foot after the other.

Don't forget to take some deep breaths while you warm up. The purpose of a good warm-up is to raise your heart rate by between 15 and 20 beats per minute and to become mentally prepared for action too.

The cool-down

Just as important as your warm-up is the cooling down stage. If you stop exercising suddenly, the muscles can become stiff and lose their flexibility.

So, whenever you've stopped doing whatever you've been doing, do a few basic stretches and movements of your choice, and then lie on the floor and circle your ankles, then hug your knees a few times (hang on in hugged position if it feels good) and then stretch out fully on the floor. Most people tend to skip this part of their schedule, but it is not only a sensible investment, it is also very relaxing.

WHAT TO DO IF YOU INJURE YOURSELF

If, in spite of your careful efforts, you know you have injured yourself, you will need to get some kind of professional help. For most people who put their back out, or damage or sprain a joint, a visit to the doctor is the first stage.

A GP may refer you to a local, probably hospital based NHS physiotherapist. For back injuries especially, most GPs will probably recommend rest for one or two days and painkillers, and then may refer you to a physiotherapist later. Some may well suggest that you seek out an alternative therapist, such as an osteopath or chiropractor (whom you will pay privately).

Physiotherapy

Physiotherapists combine exercises with massage and manipulation in order to provide relief for musculoskeletal injuries. As with any professional, you may have to try out one or two physiotherapists before you find one whose approach suits you.

But before they start any treatment, a careful diagnosis will be made to identify exactly what you've done to yourself. The physiotherapist's main tools are his or her hands. An increasing range of technological gadgetry is also available, which will help soothe and repair damaged muscles and tissues.

Ultrasound is particularly useful for sports injuries and it can be used to help encourage anti-inflammatory creams or cortisone to penetrate deep into the skin where the injury has occurred. This painless treatment involves moving the end of the ultrasound machinery over the skin, which has been coated with some transparent gel.

TENS or Transcutaneous Nerve Stimulation uses electrodes to relieve pain, usually in sessions lasting up to 20 minutes. TENS is very safe (it is also used by some women during the early stages of pain in childbirth). TENS should only be used in consultation with medical professionals, and should never be used if you have a cardiac pacemaker.

Alternative therapies

You can also try using an osteopath or chiropractor to sort out your problem if the more conventional approach has failed. These practitioners use different manipulative techniques to try and sort things out and put the body back to normal.

See page 79 of the Resources section for the addresses of the British Chiropractic Association and the General Council and Register of Osteopaths.

Sports clinics

Sometimes neither your physiotherapist nor your alternative therapist can successfully get you back into shape after an injury. In this case, it may be worth seeking out your local sports injury clinic.

You do not have to be a sportsman, or even to have sustained your injury in any sporting endeavour, in order to gain benefit from their expert knowledge of the structure of the body. Poor posture, or lifting a heavy package awkwardly, is just as likely to result in a painful injury requiring specialist attention as a genteel game of tennis on your local court or an aerobics class.

The Sports Council has a list of sports clinics throughout the UK. See page 79 in the Resources section.

BACK PAIN

Back pain is a very common problem, affecting up to half the workforce in any given year. Indeed, it is the country's number one cause of days taken off work.

A staggering 33.5 million days are lost each year, as people are rendered immobile by back pain. According to the Office of

Health Economics, back problems among the working population cost more than £1,000 million in lost production because workers have had to take time off in order to recover. And still worse than that, research by the Consumers Association shows that back problems can lead to one person in 20 having either to give up work completely or to change jobs.

What job do you do?

Your job affects your chances of developing back problems, with sedentary office workers being in the highest risk category, up there with builders and nurses and others whose work involves far more physical exertion.

People whose work involves sitting at a desk for most of the day, particularly if they are required to concentrate for long periods, may suffer from stiffness and eventual back pain, unless they take specific steps to avoid it.

So why does back pain affect sedentary workers so badly? Well, back pain is most common among those who don't exercise enough, those who are overweight and those who are not very careful about lifting heavy objects.

Given the huge costs in lost production, you would have thought that companies would be in the forefront of ordering and demanding ergonomically designed office furniture which would minimise the risks of the workers using them developing poor posture.

Fully adjustable desks and chairs can be bought readily, and although they cost more than the standard issue office furniture, the extra investment is worthwhile for everyone concerned. We are all of different heights, shapes and weights, and it is clearly absurd that a 6 foot, 13 stone man should be expected to work at a desk and on a chair similar to those that are comfortable for a 5 foot, 8 stone woman. Yet in spite of the absurdity of this, most offices make the same provision for both workers.

Standard work-surfaces, in kitchens and offices, are made to suit people of average height. If you are taller or shorter than average, and your work involves standing or sitting at such surfaces, you can expect trouble.

Similarly, desk workers who spend all day poring over papers, or staring at a screen for hours at a time, may well find that by the end of the day their shoulders are stiff or their necks hurt. They may develop a condition known as fibrositis, a short-lived muscular inflammation, which can be avoided if regular breaks are taken throughout the working day from the working area.

Almost half of all back problems are caused by people lifting heavy objects awkwardly. If your work involves lifting heavy boxes, for example, make sure that you know the correct way in which to bend and lift – otherwise let an expert move the stuff.

Sometimes the lifting is unavoidable – nurses being a prime example. Research shows that nearly one in five nurses suffers from severe backache – almost as many as those who work in heavy industry!

Are you at risk?

Taller, heavier people tend to be at the greatest risk of suffering back pain, though it can strike anyone, of any build.

Prevention is possible. Here are a few guidelines that will help you avoid backache.

Maintain your ideal bodyweight – being overweight is a major risk factor.

- **Exercise and tone muscles – especially in the abdomen.**
- **Think about your posture throughout the day, every day.**

Sitting

- Sit up, shoulders back, tummy in, bottom firmly into the back of your chair.

- Choose a chair of the right height, with a firm seat, which supports your lower back. Use a cushion if necessary in order to arch your back and force your shoulders back so that you don't slouch. The back-rest should be adjustable, and you should alter it until you feel well supported.

- Ideally, you should work at a desk with an adjustable height and experiment until you find a comfortable level. Your forearms should be at right-angles to your upper arms with the desk-top a few inches above your thighs. Very tall people should place books or solid weights under the feet of their desk in order to raise the level of the working surface. This should help them sit correctly and not slump over their work.

- Position your desk sensibly so that you do not have to keep turning round whenever people come in the room. Keep away from the glare of sunlight or you will crane your neck to avoid it whenever the sun is out. Work with your back away from draughts.

- Do not cross your legs one over the other, and ensure that your feet rest on the floor so the weight is off your thighs. If necessary, use a foot rest (or a couple of telephone directories) to support your feet.

- Don't lean forward more than you have to – your head weighs about a stone. Raise the screen if you look at a VDU so that you are looking ahead or up, rather than down.

- Keep your elbows at right angles when using a keyboard or sitting at a desk and use a document holder if you do a lot of keying in, to minimise repetitive neck movements.

- Don't sit in the same position for more than 20 minutes at a time. Get up and walk around and stretch your muscles.

Standing

Stand tall, tucking your bottom under. Imagine a piece of string attached to the top of your head, pulling it upwards. Relax your shoulders and push them back, without tensing them.

● Never slouch and try not to fold your arms as this rounds your shoulders and tips your weight forwards.

● Balance your weight evenly between both feet, and don't shift your weight from one foot to the other.

Walking

● Walk properly with your knees facing forwards and putting your heels to the ground first, using the whole foot in a rocking motion. No part of the foot should carry the whole weight of the body for more than a second.

● Wear low heels rather than high ones and make sure the straps are firm – not slingbacks or shoes that make you shuffle. You should be able to shake your foot firmly without the shoe coming off.

● Get the width of your foot measured correctly at a shoeshop. Adults think their feet stay the same size, but they can in fact change. If your shoes all feel uncomfortable, you may have gone up a size without realising it. (After childbirth, for example, women often find they go up at least a shoe size and shoe width, because the ligaments have stretched during pregnancy.)

Driving

● As with sitting, make sure that your lower back is supported. If it isn't, you can buy a special lumbar cushion or springy extra seat.

● Adjust the seat and mirror so that all the controls are within comfortable reach – people who share cars often drive in unsuitable positions for their own height, arm and leg lengths.

● Use a head-rest to support your head more comfortably, and reduce the chances of suffering a painful whiplash if you have to brake suddenly or are involved in an accident.

● Wear flat or low-heeled shoes to avoid stretching your leg muscles uncomfortably.

● Avoid bucket seats, as fitted in sporty cars, as these tend to round the backbone and spine and cause backache, especially on long or stressful journeys.

Domestic work

● If your job involves standing or sitting near worktops, make sure that these are the correct height and angle for you personally.

● Buy long-handled brushes and tools to minimise repetitive bending and stretching.

● When lifting heavy loads, avoid doing this on your own. Get someone to help, and when you lift, crouch down, knees bent, don't stoop at the waist. Get under the box and push upwards rather than stooping over and lifting towards you.

● If carrying heavy loads, make sure you are correctly balanced before you start walking.

● Take regular breaks if your work involves sitting in one position for long periods, especially if you are having to concentrate.

● Make sure that you have all the workspace you need and that you are not having to work in cramped surroundings, craning your neck or moving awkwardly to get to your papers, etc.

● Try to work near a window, with natural light. Straining to see things under the shadows caused by artificial light may cause neck and back strain, especially on the short winter days. A personal desk light will augment any overhead fluorescent lighting.

- If you use a VDU, make sure the lighting is correct and use a screen if you find you are squinting to cut out any glare. Try to use the special VDU 'workstations', which are specially, ergonomically designed for the equipment, rather than a computer on an old-fashioned table/desk.
- Use a copy-stand alongside the VDU at the same height, to avoid moving your neck up and down to look at paperwork on the desk.
- Never sit at your VDU for more than 50 minutes in every hour. Take a break to do something else, make a phone call or whatever. If your boss complains, point out that research shows that concentration is actually increased by such breaks, not decreased, and that your decision making will be enhanced also. Besides, people whose work has involved hour after hour sitting at a VDU (writers and journalists especially) are among those at the highest risk of developing repetitive strain injuries (RSI). These are not only very painful, but often involve weeks spent off work, and recently there have been several substantial compensation awards made against employers for industrial injuries.

CHAPTER SEVEN

Excuses, excuses...

Everyone's first – and most convincing – reason for not doing any form of exercise, is usually that they simply don't have the time. We all lead busy lives, but while a few people are trying to fit a 14-hour working day into every 24 hours, most of us have a fair amount of free time in any given week, if not in every single day.

Be honest. Isn't not having the time really just an excuse? We're all guilty of it. The reality is that you have to make time to do the things you really want to do, and this includes making space in your daily life for exercise. Most people, however busy they are, can find a way of doing it. Sit down, work out how to do it and then plant it in your diary.

PLANNING

This is especially important if you've got out of the habit of doing exercise. You therefore need to treat being 'active' in as organised a way as you would, say, making an appointment to have your hair cut or making a shopping list.

Once you've fitted exercise into your weekly schedule, it will be on your mind. Even if you have to change your plans as the days pass, you will be conscious of the fact that you had planned to be active and this should be sitting at the back of your mind waiting to be re-scheduled as soon as you get the next opportunity.

For example, you may have planned to play football (either with your mates or with your kids in the local park) on Saturday. The day dawns wet and miserable, or you wake up with a headache. Never mind, re-arrange your day to suit the weather and your head. But bear in mind that you've 'missed' your activity and perhaps go swimming the next day or kick a ball around the park one day after work as soon as it is dry and sunny again.

Once you start to think of exercise in the same way as you think of shopping or meeting a friend for a drink after work, you should find that it gradually starts to become part of your way of life. When you've achieved this, you've really cracked it. Unlike something that is imposed or 'one-offish', it is difficult to drop.

THE RIGHT ACTIVITY FOR YOU

Your chosen activity will depend on the kind of person you are and the kind of lifestyle you lead. Think about this carefully.

If, for example, you work with people all day and spend a lot of time in and out of meetings, you may welcome the opportunity to spend some time alone in the gym or going off on a lone bike ride. You will probably enjoy getting away from it all and disappearing on your own to work off steam and energy.

If, on the other hand, you work alone most of the time, the prospect of exercising with other people may be much more enticing. Try a group tennis coaching session (in summer) or a busy exercise class (in winter).

'Activate' your chores

If you're really short of time, you may find that you can build extra exercise into your existing and unavoidable activities. In this way, you will effectively kill two birds with one stone.

Consider your journey to work. Do you drive, or use public transport, or a mixture of the two? Is there some element of your journey where you could walk or cycle? You may even find that it takes you no more time to do this.

By the time you've driven to the station, walked from the carpark, walked along the platform, waited for the train, walked to the bus stop at the other end, caught the bus and walked from the bus stop to the office, it might have been quicker, simpler even, to cycle the whole way, door to door. If the distance is too far, then consider walking or cycling at one end or the other. You can buy an old bike, lock it to the railings and still save on bus fares.

If you're a working parent, how do you normally take the kids to or from school? By car or public transport? Could you all walk or cycle? Especially in the summer? You might have to make a bit more time – but, again, if you stop to consider the time spent stuck in traffic and looking for a parking space, the difference may be very small.

On a day-to-day basis, maybe this is impractical, but what about weekends? What about the shopping? Do you have to go by car? Could you not go by foot sometimes? Or by bike if you have one? And carry the stuff home? Obviously not the heavy stuff – but re-plan your shopping expeditions so that once a week you leave the car at home and do the whole thing the more strenuous way?

This might sound mad at first, but if you live in a town, by the time you've factored in the time spent actually getting to the supermarket carpark, the time spent driving round and round for a space, the time spent loading and unloading the shopping into the boot, you might find that it is actually quicker to do the whole thing by foot. If the energy required sounds daunting, and you usually shop in the afternoon when you are already flagging, why not switch your timetable round and get in there as soon as the supermarkets open?

KEEP A DIARY

The important thing to remember, if this is to work, is to use your diary. Work out what your chosen form of activity is going to be, and then slot it into the diary along with everything else. In this way, there is less danger of you either forgetting or dropping your best intentions when other demands intrude on your time . By all means change your plans if you have to, but don't cross out what your intentions were – just move them to another time, or even another day.

This is why exercise classes work so well for people who like to be organised rather than self-starting. Psychologically, the fact that they take place at a certain time, every week, on the same day, means that you can plan the rest of your time around them, giving structure to your week. Somehow, planning to go off to the gym, or for that bike ride, or for a brisk long walk, is infinitely off-puttable unless you have a definite time fixed when you are going to do it.

Writing things down is also very therapeutic and helps you see more clearly what you are doing and achieving and where you're heading. Below is a sample diary.

Activity diary			
	Morning	*Lunch*	*Afternoon*	*Evening*
Mon	Office	With friend	Office	Watching TV
Tues	Office	In pub	Office	At home
Wed	Office	Shopping	Office	Cinema
Thurs	Office	Sandwich in office	Office	Visit to see friends
Fri	Office	In pub	Shopping	Parents to supper
Sat	Hairdresser	At home	Tidy house	Out with friends
Sun	Supermarket	At home with friends	Gardening	Watching TV

Take a look at your diary – it may look as sedentary as this one. Now try to put something active in every day.

Book something today!

Find something that you know – or think – you'll like doing, pick up that telephone and book it *now*. Write it in your diary and then you know you will do it.

If, for example, you've settled on a summer course of tennis lessons to brush up your game, the fact that you have it to look forward to will inspire you to start thinking about getting into shape. Sort out the right clothing and footwear so you're absolutely ready to get going.

Your chosen activity may not be one that will set you on a fast lane to fitness but it will at least get you moving. And you will find that, once you've started moving, you'll soon get into a different busier frame of mind.

Scheduling

Scheduling is most important. You must work out a timetable that suits you and your current lifestyle.

If you're single but dating a regular partner, s/he will not necessarily be amused if you have arranged your life so that you are doing a workout at your local gym five nights a week and have no time left to go out socialising.

If, on the other hand, you have a family, it's no good planning time-consuming activities for weekends when you all want to be together. If you are a parent of small children, it can be very hard to justify paying, or dumping them with, someone else while you go off and do some exercise.

Similarly, it may be hard for you to get going at 6am, or 9pm, which are the only times that your partner can hold the fort while you disappear for an hour or two. There are some exercise classes that have creches attached, so investigate whether there is one near you. If all else fails, an exercise video, done either on your own or with a friend or two, is something you can do with the kids around (they might even join in!).

If you work in an office which is located close to a sports or leisure centre, you may find it much easier to join in activities there, either straight after or before work, or perhaps in your lunch hour. If there is a pool near your office, for example, a swim after a tiring day behind your desk may be just the thing to help you unwind.

What if I'm not in the mood?

This often happens and it's probably best that you don't force yourself to exercise when you really don't feel like it. Perhaps you're too tired, or you feel sluggish after a bad night and not enough sleep.

On balance, it's better to find a time that is less than ideally convenient (by making other arrangements – e.g. getting a neighbour to collect your kids from school one day) rather than force yourself to do, say, an early-morning exercise class when you are really not ready for it. Forcing yourself to fit it all in will not work and you'll end up dropping the exercise because that's the easiest thing to let go!

LOOKING FORWARD TO IT

Try not to think of exercise as a chore. Think of it rather as a treat and something to look forward to with pleasure.

Virtually everyone who takes regular exercise can tell you that not only do they enjoy doing it at the time, but afterwards they feel much better able to cope with the pressures of a busy life. Exercise sharpens the mind as well as the body and helps you to cope much better.

Too tired?

Even if you feel you are too tired, regular exercise makes you feel less tired and gives you more energy to accomplish everything else you have on your plate. It will also help you sleep better, as well as improving the quality of your sleep.

Perversely, it may seem the more active you become, the less sleep you find you will need, and the more time you will find you have to do everything else. Sluggishness creates a vicious circle in which everything becomes too much effort.

CHAPTER EIGHT

Problems and bad habits

It is no good finely tuning your body and getting into near-peak physical condition if you then go and spoil it all by sitting awkwardly all day at work, or if you commute in a stressful way to work each day and have to hit the bottle hard to unwind once you get home!

It is also no good leading the relatively stressed working life of a typical executive all week – with long heavy lunches and boozy sessions in the pub after work – only to hurl yourself round the squash court every Saturday morning for a blistering hour or two.

Fitness cannot be taken in large dollops, but must be incorporated in a balanced way into your life. Only in this way can it be healthy, rather than downright hazardous!

SMOKING

Increasingly, restaurants and offices (and other public places) are sidelining smokers so that smokers are made to feel part of an unhealthy, increasingly untolerated minority. Passive smoking is becoming an important issue and has a lot to do with non-smokers being less tolerant of those smoking around them. An increasing number of legal cases are being taken, and won, by non-smokers who have developed diseases caused by their former colleagues' smoking habits.

The simple fact is smoking can prematurely shorten your life. Remember: the smoking industry needs to recruit 300 new smokers a day to replace those whose habit has killed them.

The health risks of smoking are well known. Smoking leads to lung cancer and is a major risk factor in heart disease. For women, smoking increases the risk of cervical cancer, and smoking during pregnancy increases the risk of miscarriage and giving birth to a lower birth-weight baby.

Giving up smoking

Giving up smoking is not easy: smoking is a serious addiction. You have to really want to give up to have any chance of succeeding. Smoking is both a HABIT and an ADDICTION. You need to beat both to give up successfully. Essential steps to giving up smoking are

- **Set a date to stop.** Choose a day when you are likely to be relaxed. Get rid of all your cigarettes, ashtrays and lighters the day before.
- **Think about why you smoke.** Knowing why you smoke will help you find the reasons to stop.
- **Break the links that create the habit.** If tea and coffee or cigarettes go together, drink something different. Avoid smoky places, meet friends at home. If your hands feel empty, try and find a hobby that will keep your hands busy.
- **Get support.** Tell everyone what you are doing and why. Ask them not to offer you cigarettes.
- **Take one day at a time.** Forever seems like a long time. Stick to being a non-smoker today.
- **Expect to feel rough.** Nicotine is addictive and your body will have to get used to managing without it. You may not notice any change, but you may feel irritable and light-headed or find it hard to concentrate or sleep. These feelings are only temporary and will go with time.
- **Reward yourself.** Save your cigarette money and use the money to buy yourself a treat.

- **Don't be tempted to have just one.** Before you know it you will be a smoker again.
- **Cutting down does not work.** Stopping completely is the only way.

ALCOHOL

Moderation is the key word here. While moderate drinking seems safe, excessive drinking can lead to health problems. Drinking damages the liver, increases the risk from certain types of cancer, and alcohol is a major cause of accidents (involved in over a quarter of all road deaths and as a major factor in adult drownings). Women are more susceptible to the effects of alcohol and drinking during pregnancy is associated with stillbirth and low birth-weight babies. Long-term heavy consumption of alcohol can lead to permanent brain damage: problem solving, short term memory and co-ordination are all affected.

Safe drinking

The safe drinking levels for men and women are as follows:
- for men, 21 units a week,
- for women, 14 units a week.

Drinking more than this leads to an increasing risk: the more you drink the greater your risk from alcohol-related health problems.

Alcohol is also a source of excess calories – a pint of beer can contain up to 180 calories, a glass of wine 80 calories.

You can take steps to avoid drinking too much by following these guidelines:
- try and ignore any social pressures to drink. Don't buy rounds; you may end up drinking faster then you would normally to 'keep up' with your quota.

What is a unit?

One unit equals: 1 small glass of wine (8% alcohol by volume)

1 small glass of sherry or port (20% alcohol by volume)

1 single measure of spirits (40% alcohol by volume)

¹/₂ pint of ordinary strength lager, cider or beer (3.5% alcohol by volume)

The alcoholic strength of a drink is measured by alcohol by volume (shown on labels as 'alcohol % vol' or '%vol'). The higher the number the stronger the drink.

The above information is based on pub measures – remember when drinking at home, measures can be a lot more generous. Some beers and ciders can be a lot more alcoholic than others – so be careful.

- Try alternating one alcoholic drink for one non-alcoholic drink.
- If drinking at a special occasion or a function be aware of how often the waiter is topping up your glass. Don't be afraid to say no.
- Try to meet friends away from where alcohol is sold, e.g. at community centres, cafés or the park.

Remember, you should never drink if you are going to drive or operate machinery.

POSTURE

Most of us either have bad posture or posture that can be improved. Bad posture is a habit, which means that you walk badly, sit or slouch awkwardly and/or sleep in less than ideal conditions.

While you can be forgiven for not holding perfect positions while you are asleep, there is less excuse for your waking hours. If you permanently adopt poor posture and, at the same time, take very little exercise and allow stress to build up in your body over a period of time, you can become unbalanced and even unwell as a result.

Sitting

If your job requires you to sit for long periods, make sure that your seat is the right height for your desk and that the machines you use are all at a comfortable height or distance. Your bottom should be firmly wedged into the back of your chair, and your back well supported all the way up. Your shoulders should be relaxed and held well back, not hunched. And the lighting should be such that you do not have to squint or work at an odd angle to see what you are doing.

All of this is even more important if you have ever suffered from back or neck problems or if you get frequent headaches. It may help to keep a 'Symptoms diary' rather like your activity diary – to see if you can trace what aches and pains might be related to what work-related activities you do. Overleaf is a sample diary.

Symptoms diary

	Activity	Time	Symptom	Comment
Mon	Working at desk	Most of day	Headache	Tired/tense
Tues	Driving in traffic	Half day	Neck stiff	Stressed
Wed	Working at desk	Half day	Backache	Worked too intensely
Thurs	Driving in light traffic	All day	None	Just tired!
Fri	Doing files/ typing	All day	Backache	A lot of bending
Sat	Shopping/barbers entertaining	All day	None	Busy
Sun	Reading Sunday papers/lunch/ lazing around	All day	None	Lazy day!

Keep your diary for a few weeks, noting whenever you get a headache or other sort of pain and see if you can see a pattern emerging. You may find that you get headaches more when you are in an office all day, sitting at your desk, or alternatively that you get them when you are trying to get around in heavy traffic, or perhaps when you are rushing around all day and perhaps skipping lunch. For this reason, you might also like to note the foods and drinks that you have.

Also, note where you seem to get most of your problems. If they are work-related, you may unwittingly be suffering aggravation from noise levels or even from air pollution. The typical office is open-plan, air-conditioned, with uncontrolled noise levels and a hot stuffy atmosphere with an excess of positive ions, leading to irritability and headaches particularly among those of us who are lucky enough to be used to fresher air!

Once you have identified the possible cause of your symptoms, you can then try to alleviate matters. If your working environment is very noisy, for example, see if you can have your desk moved, or try asking about some sound insulation.

As far as the air is concerned, simply opening a window may make all the difference and you may find sitting by a window helps if it is too stuffy for you. Have the air-conditioning checked if it seems as if the air is stale. Ask if your company will install ionisers which emit negative ions (of the kind produced in thunderstorms) to make the air healthier for you. You might be able to get one at home too – they are not expensive, less than £20 these days.

Taking a break

If you do do anything for extended periods, such as sitting at a desk working and staring at a screen, it is vital to have lots of small breaks. These don't necessarily have to be coffee breaks. They might just be a question of getting up from your chair, walking around, stretching and flexing all the muscles in your body. Try rolling your shoulders, rotating your neck and shaking your arms around a bit.

Your colleagues may look a bit surprised at first, but they'll soon get used to your gyrations. Who knows, they may even copy your good habits after a while?

The same principle applies to long car journeys, especially if you get stuck in a jam. Put the handbrake on, get out and stretch all those cramped, tense muscles and limbs. This is much better than sitting hunched up and gripping the steering wheel in frustration and misery!

Don't worry about wasting time, you'll be twice as efficient either at your work, or behind the wheel, as you would have been without that break.

Useful tips

Throughout the day, try to remember the following tips. They may all seem like small things in themselves, but they will save you a lot of pain and stiffness later.

- Shoulders back and down, never rounded and hunched.
- Bottom tucked in and under and feet nicely balanced apart.
- Remember that your body was designed to keep moving, not to sit around for long periods of time. Keep moving. Even when you are stuck in traffic, you can still rotate your head, shoulders and stretch your arms, if not your legs.
- It is obviously impractical for most of us to keep moving and do our work at the same time, but it is not impossible to punctuate your daily schedule with mini-activity breaks that ensure that your muscles do not stiffen and that tension is not allowed to build up.

SLEEP

Getting the right amount of sleep is crucial as part of your overall fitness plan. This may not mean getting more sleep – indeed, you may find, on reflection, that you are sleeping too much, and that if you clipped an hour's sleep off a night, you would suffer no ill-effects. You could then raise your waking activity levels – and find that precious time to take more exercise!

Quality, rather than quantity is the key to successful sleeping habits, and while the average quota for adults is eight hours a night, there is no evidence that getting less sleep than this causes great ill-health or loss of efficiency.

How much sleep do I need?

We all tend to get obsessed with the idea that something dreadful will happen if we don't get enough sleep. Experiments have shown that humans deprived of sleep can survive for over a week without suffering from any ill-effects. You certainly don't need to worry if you miss a couple of hours here and there, with business trips or weekends away for example.

It is said that the 'thinkers' need the most sleep, while the 'doers' need the least. Perhaps active brains need more sleep than active bodies!

Two of our Prime Ministers seem to have called that view into question. Winston Churchill was once asked what he considered to be the most valuable attribute for the job of Prime Minister and he replied that it was the ability to manage on very little sleep. Margaret Thatcher was famous for her ability to manage on just five hours a night.

Most of us do not aspire to being the prime minister but we do worry if our sleep pattern starts going wrong. Most of us rush off to our GPs to ask for sleeping pills – indeed, one in ten of us takes something to get us off to sleep – making a staggering 16 million prescriptions for sleeping pills each year.

While these may help for the odd night, or the occasional period of short-lived stress – a new job, recovering after an illness, or some domestic upheaval, they are not a good long-term solution.

The most refreshing sleep

The latest thinking is that those who sleep more than nine hours a night spend more time in the dreaming sleep – which is the rapid eye-movement (REM) sleep.

This sleep is thought to be less refreshing than the orthodox or non-dreaming sleep, people who manage on less sleep tend to have deep orthodox sleep, with fewer dreams and disturbed nights.

We apparently need more of the orthodox sleep than the REM sleep. If we miss out on the non-dreaming sleep, we tend to become depressed or lethargic. Whereas if we miss out on dreaming sleep, we tend to become more irritable.

During the night, we move from one kind of sleep to the other, starting off with deep orthodox sleep, which usually comprises about three-quarters of the night's total sleep. Most of us take about 15 minutes to drop off, and as we do so blood pressure, heart-rate and body-temperature all fall. Most of us don't start dreaming for about an hour and a half, moving into the lighter REM sleep phase.

Physically, we burn fewer calories when we are asleep than when we are awake, so if you can shorten the time spent asleep, even by a small amount, graduating to a larger amount, you can make your calorific burn-up much higher by this relatively simple (and painless) method!

Getting a good night's sleep

If you have sleep problems, lack of exercise may be the reason. It often is.

Stepping up your level of activity will make you more physically tired and ready for sleep. Physical tiredness also helps to overcome the kind of anxiety that keeps you awake at night, tossing and turning and churning ideas over in your head.

As adults, we forget to 'wind down' as we were taught as children. Instead of taking a long soak in the bath, we eat indigestible meals, late in the evening, drink tea and coffee with caffeine and drink alcohol. No wonder that when we try to fall asleep our minds are still whizzing round and round!

Useful tips

Here are some useful tips that will help you ensure a good night's sleep.

- Cut down on caffeinated drinks – have no more than three cups of real coffee during the day. Remember that tea contains caffeine also, though in lower doses than coffee, so do fizzy drinks like Cola.
- Don't drink any caffeinated drinks late in the day.
- Drink de-caffeinated brews if you can't possibly cut down.
- Drink a milky drink before bed as milk contains tryptophan, a substance that promotes sleep.
- Unwind by reading or listening to relaxing music or the radio. Talking books are wonderfully soporific!
- Have a warm bath rather than a shower. The first relaxes, the other stimulates!
- If you are still awake after 15 minutes, get up and do something that you have been putting off. If your mind is 'whizzing', write a list of everything you have to do in the morning and then try again.
- Don't eat gaseous or very rich foods late at night, which will keep you and your stomach 'awake'. Avoid beans, nuts, fruit and raw vegetables.
- Don't panic if you can't sleep. Regard it as a bonus that you are not as tired as you thought and use the time to catch up on some reading or writing letters.
- Do some exercises, either gentle ones on the floor, or more vigorous ones if you are feeling tense and un-relaxed.

MINOR HEALTH PROBLEMS

Are you experiencing minor, but irritating health problems? Sometimes we go through phases in our life when our sleep is disturbed or we keep getting one cold after another, or suffer endless headaches.

Clearly something is wrong but the symptoms are not serious enough in themselves to warrant a trip to the doctor for a course of medicine. But why are you feeling run down? Is work proving stressful? Perhaps your life is unbalanced? Perhaps you need to get more support – either at home or at work or both. Have you taken on too much? Perhaps you should take a good hard look at your workload and see if there is anything you can delegate.

Conclusions

Being fit does not necessarily mean being healthy. Just because you can run up to your office on the fifth floor when the lift is out of order, does not necessarily mean you are in perfect working order – especially if you drink heavily every night after work and/or habitually consume large high cholesterol business lunches. Nor does hurling yourself around a squash court once or twice a week mean that you are necessarily going to avoid a heart attack!

If your lungs and heart are strong, this means that you are fit in a technical sense, but having an overall healthy approach to life will gain you more 'brownie points' in general health terms, and help ensure you never see the inside of an intensive-care ward (through any non-accidental fault of your own, at any rate!).

THE CHOICE IS YOURS

Being healthily fit is within your power. It is not a gift naturally bestowed at birth to a chosen few. Being unfit is also a choice – an unthinking one for most people and an avoidable one.

Obviously, from a safety point of view, sitting and relaxing in your armchair is one way of making sure that you stay alive. For an hour at a time, this is fine... and also for an occasional evening. But as a way of life it is bad news, and if your life has become too sedentary, now is the time to resolve to do something about it.

Most of us lead such busy lives that at the end of the working day, all we can contemplate is collapsing into bed, or that armchair in front of the telly. While our idea of a good night out is a slap-up meal, washed down with a couple of bottles of decent plonk. But as a way of life, sooner or later you slip into a lower gear, then a lower one still, until everything starts to feel like too much of a physical effort.

Staying fit for work needn't mean signing up for your local football club, nor joining an expensive health club... all you need to do is to find two or three ways to put more activity into your life on a regular, week-in, week-out basis. Organise yourself into a more active routine. It is a question of balance, not of extremes. Taking up a short-lived, vigorous, heart-thumping, sweat-dripping exercise regime is about as sensible as going on a starvation diet – and likely to be about as successful.

Don't make yourself a slave to exercise. If you don't feel 100%, don't force yourself to do a workout, take a bike-ride or whatever. If you're not in the mood, you won't enjoy it, and if you're under-par anyway, with a headache or a bad cold, you'll make yourself feel worse rather than better.

MODERATION IN ALL THINGS...

Everyone knows the rules by now for a healthy way of life. Eat a balanced nutritious diet, keep your consumption of alcohol to a reasonable level, and don't smoke. And we hope that this book has added a fourth dimension to your life – make physical activity a regular part of your routine.

None of those things – including exercise – should be done to excess. Balance and moderation are the key words in everything.

Some people get away with smoking, drinking and eating to excess all their lives and taking far too little exercise. We all know people who do. Good luck to them if they can get away with it... for as long as they do.

Statistically though, we also know that if we indulge in these nasty habits willy-nilly, sooner or later they will catch up with us. We will fall ill and life will become, at the very least, less enjoyable, and at worst, drastically shortened.

Doctors and medicine can only patch us up, they cannot make us healthy in the first place. The onus is on each of us to make the most of the knowledge we have, and the increasing amounts of time at our disposal, to make the most of life, without burning out too soon.

After all, it is your body. You only have one, and you only have one life. Treat your body with respect. Look after it and you will be rewarded through the rest of your life.

Resources

BIBLIOGRAPHY

Archer, M. (1988) *Fit for Business*, Mercury Business Paperbacks.

Ashton, D. (1993) *The 12 Week Executive Health Plan*, Kogan Page.

Baum, G. (1991) *Aquarobics: Working Out in Water*, Arrow.

Cannon G. and Einzig, H. (1983) *Dieting Makes You Fat*, Century.

Clark, J. (1992) *Full Life Fitness*, Human Kinetics Publishers (USA).

The Complete Manual of Fitness and Wellbeing (1984) Readers Digest.

Connolly, C. and Einzig, H. (1986) *Fitness Jungle*, Century.

Fiske, M. (1979) *Middle Age – The Prime of Life*, Harper and Rowe.

Gavin, J. (1992) *The Exercise Habit*, Human Kinetics Publishers (USA).

Gillie, O. (1984) *The Sunday Times ABC Diet and Body Plan*, Hutchinson.

Goodsell, A. (1994) *Your Personal Trainer*, Boxtree.

Hislop, B. (1993) *The Body Breakthrough*, Vermillion.

Jones, G. (1988) *Fit to Manage*, Thorsons.

Lynch, B. (1991) *The BBC Healthcheck*, BBC Books.

Melpomene Institute (1991) *The Bodywise Woman*, Human Kinetics Publishers (USA).

O'Brien, P. (1993) *Fit to Work*, Sheldon Press.

Pollitt, D. (1990) *Lifeguide*, Boxtree.

Pontefract, R. (1979) *Feel Fit, Come Alive*, Oxford University Press.

The Pritkin Programme for Diet/Exercise (1979) Grosset and Dunlap.

Ripley, A. and Ferris, L. (1991) *Forty Plus – Use it or Lose it*, Stanley Paul.

Scala, J. and Jacques, B. (1991) *Look Young, Feel Better*, Piatkus (USA).

Schwarzenegger, A. (1993) *Arnold's Fitness Programme for Kids*, Vermillion.

Scully, P. (1991) *Modern Gym Fitness: The Complete Course*, Guinness.

Thomas, D. and Rippee, N. (1992) *Is Your Aerobics Class Killing You?*, Capella Books (USA).

Tysoe, M. (1988) *All This and Work Too*, Fontana.

Wilburn, M. (1993) *Starbound*, Orion.

Wilmore, J. (1986) *Sensible Fitness*, Leisure Press (USA).

Wright, B. (1986) *Ease and Disease*, Longman.

Youngson, R. M. (1988) *The Daily Telegraph: The Healthy Executive*, Telegraph Publications.

USEFUL ADDRESSES

*** The British Chiropractic
Association**
29 Whitley Street
Reading, Berkshire RG2 0EG
01734 757 557

*** The General Council and
Register of Osteopaths**
56 London Street
Reading, Berkshire RG1 4SQ
01734 576 585

** For an SAE they will send you a
list of practitioners in your area.*

**Physical Education
Association**
Francis House
Francis Street
London SW1P 1DE
0171 828 9229

Sports Council
16 Upper Woburn Place
London WC1H 0QP
0171 388 1277

YMCA (National Council)
640 Forest Road
London E17 3DZ
0181 520 5599

Other titles in the **LIFE QUALITY MANAGEMENT SERIES**

BEATING STRESS AT WORK

Anne Woodham

A no-nonsense handbook on the causes and consequences of stress and how you can make positive changes to avoid or control it. BEATING STRESS AT WORK examines the various pressures on you, including performance pressures and deadlines, personal relationships, and your working and home environments.

07521 0168 4

£5.99

SURVIVING AT WORK

Dr Carol Cooper

An essential guide to surviving the hazards of work and staying fit, healthy and on top of your job. This helpful book looks at the working environment, and examines dangers like repetitive strain injury, passive smoking and sexual harassment.

0 7521 0166 8

£5.99

EATING WELL AT WORK

Miriam Polunin

A straightforward plan to help you keep fit and healthy despite rushed breakfasts, sinful snacks, heavy lunches and after-work drinks. The book examines what you eat during the working day, asks what food you could avoid or eat less of, and looks at when tea, coffee and alcohol can become a problem.

0 7521 0169 2

£5.99

The Life Quality Management titles are available from all good bookshops. Alternatively, use the form below to order your copies.

ORDER FORM

Please send me....... copies of

☐ **BEATING STRESS AT WORK**
0 7521 0168 4 @£5.99

☐ **SURVIVING AT WORK**
0 7521 0166 8 @£5.99

☐ **EATING WELL AT WORK**
0 7521 0169 2 @£5.99

☐ **STAYING FIT AT WORK**
0 7521 0167 6 @£5.99

Postage and packing
(80p for first copy £1.30
for two or more copies)

Total

Name:

Address:

Postcode

☐ I enclose a cheque made payable to Health Education Authority

☐ Please debit my credit card

ACCESS/VISA number

Expiry date ☐☐ / ☐☐   Signature _____

Send to:
CUSTOMER SERVICES DEPARTMENT,
Marston Book Services, PO Box 87, Osney Mead Industrial Estate, Oxford OX2 ODT